CONQUER DEPRESSION
WITHOUT
MEDICATION

A No-drug Approach to Depression and Anxiety

SMITH FORD

TABLE OF CONTENTS

INTRODUCTION

Depression is a frequent mental health problem that results in a lingering melancholy as well as changes in thinking, sleeping, eating, and acting. It can also be characterized as having poor self-esteem or remorse and having trouble enjoying life. When depressed, a person frequently exhibits several of the following signs and symptoms: sadness, hopelessness, or pessimism; diminished self-worth and increased self-depreciation; a decrease or loss of enjoyment in routine activities; diminished energy and vitality; slowness of thought or action; loss of appetite; and disturbed or unrestful sleep.

Simple sadness or mourning, which are acceptable emotional reactions to the loss of loved ones or items, are not the same as depression. When there are obvious reasons for a person to feel unhappy, depression is thought to be present if the gloomy mood is too protracted or severe in comparison to the triggering event. The division of depression into various categories is based on differences in the duration of depression, the circumstances under which it occurs, and a few other criteria. Bipolar disorder, major depressive disorder (clinical depression), persistent depressive disorder, and seasonal affective disorder are a few examples of distinct types of depression.

Even before the time of the ancient Greek physician Hippocrates, who dubbed it melancholia, physicians have been describing depression, which is likely the most prevalent psychiatric complaint. The disorder's progression might be moderate or severe, acute or chronic, and it varies greatly from person to person. Depression can linger for up to four months if left untreated. Women are twice as likely as males to experience depression. Although it can happen at any age, the average onset age is in the 20s.

Several factors can contribute to depression. Unfavorable life experiences can make someone more susceptible to depression or start a depressive episode. Depressive symptoms are produced and maintained in part by negative thoughts about oneself and the outside environment. Nonetheless, it appears that both psychological and physiological pathways are significant culprits;The primary physiological reason, in particular norepinephrine and serotonin, appears to be the improper regulation of one or more naturally occurring neurotransmitters in the brain. Some sufferers of depression are thought to have lower levels or less activity of these substances in the brain, which may be the root of their melancholy mood.

My Experience With Depression
A recovery tale is a complicated thing. It has numerous beginnings but no definitive finale. There is a lot more inaction than action, and the most of the drama and struggle occurs internally. Much of the time, the main figure stays hidden in the shadows, making it impossible to even see what's happening.

I first became depressed when I was about 8 years old. There are pictures of me wearing the worn-out brown jacket that I preferred to wear. My mother took some really lovely pictures, and several of them have me in gloomy shadows, looking as depressed as I possibly could.

She needed to focus about her own sadness. My typical memory of her at that time is of a couch-bound mother who frequently took naps. She diagnosed her sleep disorder as sleepkophasia, a term I have never been able to locate in a dictionary. After resting down for a while, snap! Totally sleeping In those days, no one brought up odd emotional issues or mental disease. On occasion, my parents described someone suffering a nervous breakdown as if they had passed away. There was no indication that my mother, much less me, needed assistance. Since I was a star student, independent, and impressive to professors for being so mature, no one worried about me.

The onset of migraines and growing levels of anxiety about school followed. I skipped numerous days, felt guilty as though I were pretending, and became fixated on all of my shortcomings. I was alone in my room for a long time. All Depression disappeared during my teen years. Emotions could be harmful. I couldn't possibly add to the barrage of irate and aggressive ones that were trembling the house. I therefore suppressed my emotions even more than I did when I was younger.

Nothing both within my house and outside of it bothered me. I showed almost no sign of reaction to anything, even while churning with fear and anguish.

When I finally cracked in my 20s, torrents of depression, anxiety, terror, obsessive love, and rage came pouring out. I visited a psychiatrist after having a panic episode for a week. In a three-hour marathon session, he assisted me in connecting my panic to terrifying incidents in my personal history. I was instantly healed, but I never saw him again. To do more would have been premature.

During a second crisis a few years later, I was finally able to see a psychiatrist again and had my first experience with Elavil. Yet, I was unsure of what it was. I took a stimulant in the morning to get me going and a sleep aid at night. I just used it briefly, got over the crisis, and kept going to therapy. For the following eight years, I continued to see psychiatrists in various places. Yet nobody brought up despair.

In a letter to the draft board during the Vietnam War, a psychiatrist used the term to describe my problem for the first time. Yet, I didn't receive care for that issue. In those days, therapy was still done in the Freudian tradition and focused mostly on family dynamics and conflict. Going deeper was facilitated by depression. Exploring the history helped me in many ways and was a huge help in understanding the difficulties of the present. Yet, depression persisted in various forms and returned frequently throughout the following few decades. I experienced ups and downs related to marriage, having kids, and a few different occupations, yet there were also incredibly joyful and prosperous periods.

My wife eventually asked that I seek treatment after my depression got to the point where it was too disruptive. So I did in the end. The 1990s were at hand. I began a twelve-year tour of medications that didn't accomplish very much once Prozac became available. Therapy didn't help either, despite the fact that two psychiatrists had helped me recognize some of my more harmful behavioral tendencies. Every aspect of my life was impacted by depression, making it more and more difficult to maintain a job and a family. The medications seemed to do nothing but numb my emotions, leaving me feeling removed from everyone and unaffected by stress. That was similar to having the pain signals muted. My body or brain no longer gave any indication that something might be wrong. Although I was "OK," my relationships and job continued to fail.

Strangely, despite having lived with depression for so many years, I didn't have a lot of knowledge about it. I initially believed that the issue was solely related to my low mood, lack of energy, and lack of motivation. As things deteriorated, I eventually began to read extensively about it.

When I discovered the full extent of depression and how ubiquitous it might be across the body and mind, I was astounded. I at last had a clear, complete understanding of what depression was.

That was a significant development since it allowed me to finally consider the likelihood of improving. I could see that I wasn't inherently useless, that there were causes for my inability to concentrate, and that this sickness was also to blame for the regular slurring of my speech and thought processes. After all, perhaps the proper care could result in important adjustments.

Yet there were still hazards up ahead. I developed an obsession with the notion that depression is a neurological condition. I researched various types of depression, as well as neuroscience and countless other topics. That was a wise move, but after a while I found myself focusing more on the word "Depression" than the specifics of my personal case of the sickness.

I questioned how many diagnostic subgroups I fell under. I most definitely had one or more anxiety problems. Maybe bipolar II is more appropriate for me than major depressive illness. How does dissociation fit in? I interpreted the research study's conclusions as a proclamation of my doom.

Knowing I had a "genuine" disease was consoling. I could not only refute any doubters on the reality of depression. I also had the residual uncertainty that I had any problems as a weapon against my internalized stigma. I had considered the possibility that I was faking my illness in order to escape reality and hide my own frailty. Here was evidence that my brain's chemistry, not my imagination, was what was causing my despair.

Neurobiology was completely out of my hands. I was unable to recover on my own. I had to be treated with medicine or other methods, such as ECT, by doctors. That meant that instead of placing my hopes in my own ability to improve, I was placing them in them.

I became certain that depression would never go away when the medications didn't help. The future was lost hope. My life would keep getting worse. Could it possibly result in suicide, as it did for some of my friends?

Fortunately, when I gained more knowledge, I paid attention to the professionals who had a far larger understanding of the reasons of the sickness. I understood from Mitcher Freed's review of the studies on depression that factors that may contribute to the condition include genetics, family history, traumatic experiences, stress, and the malfunction of numerous bodily systems. No one was able to isolate a single cause or reduce it to a handful of neurotransmitters.

So I went back to the beginning and paid much closer attention to the specific symptoms I was experiencing. I studied the small nuances of daily life and realized that I had to take the initiative in my own healing. When it had any effect at all, medication performed a small part in easing the worst symptoms. I was able to work on the emotional and relationship effects and try to straighten out the aspects of my life I had some control over because of that small sense of relief.

I was adamant about ending the futility of depression. I resumed my psychotherapy and also explored a variety of self-help techniques. Many of them failed completely, yet despite setbacks, something inside of me drove me to keep trying.
Because I know that the loneliness will pass and that I can talk myself out of feeling lonely when I am not actually alone, I push myself to spend more time with my friends.

I consume all things swoon-worthy. I play along by pretending to be one of the characters, which causes me to experience their emotions rather than my own (or preventing myself from feeling). I sing along to Taylor Swift from the past. Because what could be more lovely than a summer romance involving Chevy trucks and Tim McGraw in a little country town? And even though I occasionally let my homework slide, I always force myself to put in some effort. In essence, I make myself live my life because, well, it's my life and I don't want to spend it feeling lonely when I'm not and numb when I might be amazing. Because of my depression, I do experience such feelings far more frequently than I would like, yet I still have to deal with them.

I will always experience depression since it is an illness.

I am who I am and my depression is a part of that.

Most importantly, I want to live this life since I only have one to live. Even if at times my despair makes me want to end my life, I stubbornly refuse.

My attempt to write about my experience with depression was one of the most significant ones. One of the ways I learn new things is by writing, but for years I had avoided doing it due to a strong fear. I now see that the underlying cause of my impasse was my attempt to write about topics other than despair. Writing came effortlessly after I was able to tackle that head-on.

The ideal media turned out to be blogging. Even when I felt miserable, it was bearable. I received a kind of support from the internet depression community that I had never experienced before. Leaving my high-stress job, which I was doing less and less successfully, was another crucial move. A profound sensation of vigor was restored when that ongoing stress was lifted. Following all of this, recuperation eventually began. I was caught off guard by it, and for a while I had my doubts that it would endure. But deep down, something had shifted. I started to believe in myself once more, and the inner feeling of worthlessness vanished.

I had discovered a genuinely fulfilling reason for writing, as well as the motivation and humor to do what I wanted to do. I was able to reclaim my consciousness and emotional presence so that I could rejoin my family as the visible father and husband.

Setbacks occur, as anyone who has struggled with depression their entire life will attest to. No easy happy conclusion exists. Yet if you're fortunate, an inner change takes place, and the new normal is a good existence as opposed to depression.

Considering that I am the author of my own life, I prefer to use a semicolon rather than a period whenever my melancholy urges me to do otherwise.

Hence, my depression impacts my life in this manner. That's how I handle it. I will, whether you like it or not.

CHAPTER ONE

SYMPTOMS

You might only experience depression once in your lifetime, most people experience many bouts.

During these episodes, symptoms can include any of the following and may last for the majority of the day:

- Sadness, tears, emptiness, or a sense of futility

- Irrational behavior, irritation, or frustration, especially about trivial issues

- Loss of enjoyment or interest in the majority of everyday activities, including sex, hobbies, and sports

- Sleep disorders, such as insomnia or excessive sleeping

- Due to fatigue and a lack of energy, even simple tasks need more effort.

- Weight loss and decreased appetite, or weight gain and increased desires for food

- A feeling of unease, anxiety, or worry

- Sluggish speech, posture, or other body movements

- Feelings of guilt or worthlessness, a fixation on mistakes made in the past, or self-blame

- Problems with memory, concentration, decision-making

- Thoughts of suicide, death, or other suicidal behavior on a regular basis or repeatedly

- Undiagnosed physical issues like headaches or back pain

Many depressed individuals typically experience symptoms that are severe enough to interfere with daily activities including job, school, social interactions, or interpersonal relationships.

Some people may experience widespread misery or unhappiness without truly understanding why.

Depression in children and Teenagers

Although there may be some distinctions, the typical signs and symptoms of depression in adolescents and teenagers are comparable to those in adults.

Depression in young children might manifest as:
- melancholy

- impatience,

- clinginess

- concern

- aches and pains

- refusal to attend school

- underweight

Teens may experience symptoms such as :

- sadness

- irritability

- feeling down and unworthy

- anger

- poor performance or poor attendance at school

- feeling misunderstood and overly sensitive

- using alcohol or drugs recreationally

- eating excessively

- engaging in self-harm

- losing interest in routine activities

- avoiding social interaction

Depression in Older Adults

Depression is never to be taken lightly because it is not a typical aspect of aging. However, older persons with depression frequently go undetected and untreated, and they may be hesitant to seek help.

Older persons may experience various or less noticeable signs of depression, such as:

- memory issues or character alterations

- physical discomfort

- Symptoms of exhaustion

- anorexia

- insomnia

- loss of desire in sex that are not brought on by a disease or medication

- Often preferring to stay in rather than leave the house to interact with others or try new things

- Especially with elderly men, suicidal thoughts or feelings

CHAPTER TWO

CAUSES OF DEPRESSION

Depression can have many different causes. It has numerous triggers and a wide range of potential causes.

A traumatic or stressful life event, such as a death in the family, a divorce, a sickness, a layoff, or concerns about one's career or finances, may be the culprit for some people.

Depression frequently results from a combination of many reasons. As an illustration, you might be depressed after being ill and then go through a painful incident, like losing a loved one.

Individuals frequently discuss a "downward cycle' of circumstances that results in depression. For instance, if your relationship with your partner fails, you may feel depressed, stop seeing your friends and family, and begin drinking more. All of these may worsen your symptoms and lead to sadness.

However, some research have indicated that depression is more prevalent in older persons and in those who experience challenging social and economic conditions.

Tense Situations
Most people need some time to adjust to traumatic situations like losing a loved one or ending a relationship. When these stressful situations arise, cutting off contact with friends and family and attempting to solve your problems alone increases your risk of developing depression.

Personality

If you exhibit certain personality qualities, such as poor self-esteem or excessive self-criticism, you may be more prone to depression. Your genes from your parents, your early experiences, or both may be to blame for this.

Family Background

It is more likely that you will experience depression if someone in your family—such as a father, sister, or brother—has experienced it in the past. Family history is frequently connected to depression. Those who have depressed family members are more likely to experience depression themselves, despite the fact that precise genetic correlations have not been identified.

Having a baby

After giving birth, some women are especially susceptible to depression. Postnatal depression may result from the hormonal and physical changes, in addition to the extra burden of a new life.

Loneliness

Your chance of developing depression may increase if you experience feelings of isolation brought on by things like cutting off contact with friends and relatives.

Drugs and alcohol

Depression is frequently brought on by medications, drug and alcohol dependence, and other factors. After beginning a new drug, a patient could experience depression. Alcohol and recreational drug addiction can exacerbate the signs and symptoms of depression.

Some people turn to excessive alcohol or drug use as a coping mechanism when life becomes difficult. Depression may spiral as a result of this.

Although marijuana can help you unwind, there is evidence that it can also worsen depression, especially in youth.

Using alcohol to "drown your sorrows" is likewise not advised. Drinking alters brain chemistry, which raises the danger of depression.

Illness
If you suffer from a chronic or life-threatening ailment, such as cancer or coronary heart disease, you may be more likely to experience depression.

Depression is frequently underdiagnosed as being caused by head injuries. Emotional issues and mood swings may be brought on by a major brain injury.

Some people may experience immune system issues that lead to hypothyroidism, which is an underactive thyroid. Rarely, a mild head injury can harm the pituitary gland, a pea-sized gland at the base of the brain that generates hormones that stimulate the thyroid.

This can result in a variety of symptoms, including acute exhaustion and a loss of libido (loss of desire in sex), which can then create sadness.

Depressive episodes can be brought on by the lived experience of physical or mental abuse, sorrow, or other traumatic experiences.
Depression can be brought on by persistent medical conditions and physically crippling injuries. This is why mental health providers frequently link treating depression with a patient's overall medical care.

Some people are more prone to mental tension and bad thoughts due to their characteristics. Depression will also impact people more severely if they have low self-esteem and are perfectionists.
In addition to the aforementioned variables, increasingly frequent life occurrences including loneliness, job loss, a breakup or divorce, and bereavement are some of the very modern causes of depression.

Let's learn as a culture how to address anxiety and depression more effectively without using drugs.

Perhaps depression is a natural part of being human. That does not imply that we cannot heal or that medication is always necessary. There are natural approaches that can help alleviate depression without medicine or antidepressants, such as diet, exercise, and meditation.

Rapid eye movement (REM) sleep disorders and depression are related. Neurons in the amygdala, a part of the brain thought to be important in controlling REM sleep, project into the brainstem. In certain sad people, the amygdala may be enlarged, hyperactive, or otherwise malfunctioning because it is also connected to processing unfavorable ideas.

The importance of these correlations has to be determined, but the linkage between depression, disturbed REM sleep, and amygdala abnormalities has opened up new paths for investigation into the neurobiology and management of depression. According to research, physical activity may help reduce a person's risk of acquiring depression because it is linked to depression. Comparatively to those who do not exercise, those who exercise frequently report having better mental health and are less likely to experience depression.

CHAPTER THREE

TYPES OF DEPRESSION

The three main kinds of depression are
- bipolar disorder,
- major depressive disorder
- persistent depressive disorder

Bipolar disorder is characterized by alternating episodes of depression and mania (an abnormal elevation of mood) or hypomania (a distinct elevation of mood that is not necessarily abnormal). Major depressive illness is defined by severe symptoms that interfere with a person's daily activities, frequently affecting the person's ability to enjoy life, sleep, eat, or work. Major depressive episodes can strike anyone at any age, and they might happen only once or repeatedly over the course of a person's life. A major depressive episode may occasionally accompany the symptoms of persistent depressive illness, which remain for two years or longer.

Additional forms of depression include psychotic depression, seasonal affective disorder, and postpartum depression, each of which appears under particular conditions. Women experience postpartum depression in the time after giving birth. Anxiety, a lack of interest in raising the child, and emotions of despair, helplessness, or inadequacy are other symptoms. The "baby blues," a frequent ailment among women after childbirth that often entails mood fluctuations, feelings of sadness, and weeping fits, are shorter-lived and less severe than postpartum depression.

In the context of psychosis, which can include symptoms of delusion, hallucination, or paranoia, psychotic depression develops. The hallmark of seasonal affective disorder is the onset of depressed symptoms in the fall and winter, which are relieved by more exposure to sunlight in the spring and summer.

CHAPTER FOUR

TREATING DEPRESSION WITHOUT MEDICATION

The degree and pattern of depression cycles determine the usual treatment strategies for depression. In order to determine the intensity and subtype of your depression, a doctor's mental evaluation is typically the first step in receiving standard treatment. Moreover, routine testing like hemograms, cholesterol analyses, and blood sugar checks will be performed. An extensive treatment plan is created after a medical examination of all this data.

The main focus of the treatment strategy will frequently be psychological therapies such cognitive behavioral therapy, behavioral activation, and interpersonal psychotherapy. Is there just one main factor that contributes to depression? It's challenging

A mental health crises like depression cannot be solely attributed to one cause. Popular culture may attribute negative thinking or childhood trauma, but the truth is considerably more nuanced. The WHO claims that a "complex combination of social, psychological, and biological variables" causes depression.

Combination strategies are the most effective technique to combat depression. Why not try out a few of the strategies given here if you are having trouble deciding where to start and see what works for you? You can find out what treatments, such as tDCS, medication, or possibly both, will help you lessen your depression symptoms by committing to a few practices. Keep in mind that there is no one proven, effective method for treating depression. What functions best for you will depend on your experience and the particular chemical balance in your brain.

We are on your side. In the event that you encounter depressive symptoms, always speak with your doctor. Depending on how severe your problem is, medication might be advised, at least initially.. Otherwise, you might be able to use these non-drug methods to control and even stop depressive episodes.

Some of the symptoms of depression can be treated in a variety of ways without the use of prescription drugs. If you suffer from depression, you might want to try treating it without medication or as a supplement to your antidepressant. If so, look over these natural options and then discuss with your doctor which ones might be appropriate for your treatment plan.

This book talks about several all-natural remedies for depression, such as dietary adjustments and supplements. It also discusses additional tactics you may use, such improving your home environment or engaging in mindfulness exercises.

Natural Depression Treatments
You might feel powerless if you're depressed. There are many things you may do on your own to fight back, in addition to treatment and perhaps medicine. Natural depression therapies include altering your physical activity, manner of living, and even your way of thinking.

You can start feeling better right away by using these suggestions.

Establish a routine

You need a routine if you're depressed because depression can make life unstructured. The days blend into one another. An easy daily routine can assist you in getting back on track.

Moreover, melancholy symptoms might make it challenging to follow a schedule, Nonetheless, evidence indicates that maintaining a routine may be important for mental wellness. When you are struggling with depression, stress, or anxiety, keeping a routine can help you maintain a sense of normalcy and stability.

On the other hand, not having a regular routine can make you feel more stressed, overwhelmed, and unable to concentrate. Therefore make an effort to have a plan that includes both plenty of time for self-care and the essential tasks you need to complete.

Establish objectives.

When you're depressed, you might think there's nothing you can do. You start to feel worse about yourself as a result. Make daily goals for yourself in order to push back.

Start off very modestly. Set a realistic goal for yourself, such as doing the dishes every other day.

You can increase the difficulty of your daily goals as you begin to feel better.

Exercise

Endorphins, which are feel-good compounds, are momentarily increased. Those with depression might potentially benefit over the long run from it. Frequent physical activity appears to stimulate the brain to positively remodel itself. What level of workout is required? To receive a benefit, you don't have to run marathons. Even just a few weekly walks can be beneficial. Depression can be treated without medicine with exercise. Regular exercise must be mentioned for a piece on evidence-based depression therapies to be considered complete.

Exercise is a potent, all-natural treatment for depression that is as effective as both medications and psychotherapy.

Think about the chemistry: when you exercise, your body releases substances called endorphins. In addition to making us "feel good," endorphins also function as an analgesic and lessen our perception of pain.

Moreover, exercise promotes brain plasticity. Physical activity increases neuroplasticity in adults who are not depressed and improves the clinical symptoms of major depressive illness, according to a 2020 study from Germany.

Why does mental exercise feel so good?

How is it that something as basic as walking can be so good for the brain and just as helpful for alleviating depression symptoms as medication? According to neuroscientists, your brain releases neurotransmitters like dopamine and serotonin when you exercise. You experience pleasure and happiness thanks to these molecules. Yet the benefits of working up a sweat aren't only immediate.
Long-term, exercise really produces new brain cells, strengthening your brain's resistance to depression and other disorders because of all that greater flexibility.

How much exercise is therefore necessary to alleviate depression symptoms?

Is stretching sufficient to combat sadness, or do you also require frequent spin classes? The solution lies somewhere in the middle. Frequent walking is a fantastic method for managing depressed symptoms without the need of drugs. The following is the exact recipe provided by Dr. Wendy Suzuki, professor of neural science and psychology at New York University:

a 30- to 40-minute workout It just takes 3–4 sessions each week to overcome depression.

More than that is not necessary, although it is crucial to work up a sweat. You could suffer the following negative consequences if you're new to exercising: skin flushing, heart racing and heavy breathing. Not to worry. This is merely a greeting from your sympathetic nervous system; it is not an allergy of any kind. Many people have trouble exercising, particularly those who are depressed. If you're just getting started, try to be modest.

According to all available information, frequency and consistency are more crucial than initial intensity. That example, every time you go outside, add a few minutes and take a 10-minute walk rather than a 30-minute jog. A half-hour or so of low-intensity action each day has been found to be useful in enhancing mood and quality of life, so getting more exercise doesn't need imply training for a marathon. 12 Better still, do it outside. Particularly restorative are sunlight and fresh air are healing for dealing with a special form of depression known as seasonal affective disorder (SAD).

Although studies have shown that regular exercise can help prevent and treat depression,13 it can be challenging to develop a regular exercise routine when you're feeling down. You might feel too worn out to get up and move around because of a lack of energy and a bad attitude.

You might try the following to maintain your habit:

At least a few times every week, go for a stroll with a loved one or engage in some other sort of physical activity. Not only can a friend's support get you started on a regimen, but it may also keep those social ties alive when you're feeling depressed.
Think about the advantages. Starting is difficult, but finishing it is something that will help you feel better in the long term.

Begin by going for short daily walks, then work your way up to longer ones. Strong evidence supports the idea that regular exercise of any form is one of the best antidepressants. It can stop mild depression from turning into a more severe form of depression, in addition to helping to keep your current mental state from getting worse. Exercise helps to increase energy levels, enhance sleep quality, and lessen anxiety symptoms.

Exercises reduces depression by boosting endorphins, which are euphoric, natural substances. According to some study, aerobic exercise may have a particularly potent antidepressant impact. In a study on depression and anxiety, it was discovered that patients with significant depression who exercised for an average of 45 minutes three days a week for three months experienced a reduction in their symptoms and for at least two months experienced a greater antidepressant effect compared with those who did minimal exercise.

Yet any kind of exercise, no matter how intense, is beneficial. Concentrate on what you enjoy doing since mobility is important. People in civilizations with the lowest rates of depression and the highest quality of life don't frequent gyms; instead, they exercise a lot during the course of the day. Simple forms of exercise include going for a daily stroll, taking care of your garden, or working on home improvement tasks.

Getting your body moving can help you overcome depression.

Diet as depression treatment

Altering your food is another another medication-free depression therapy option.

There isn't a magic food that will make you happy again. But you should keep an eye on your diet. Gaining control over your eating will improve your mood if depression causes you to overeat.

There is evidence that eating foods high in folic acid and omega-3 fatty acids, such as spinach and avocado, may help treat depression, however nothing is conclusive.

According to research, those who consume a lot of red meat, added sugars, high-fat dairy products, fried foods, and creamy sauces are more likely than others to have depression symptoms and low moods.

This implies that a depressed mood is caused by sugar and fat. Also, it implies that a dinner at the closest fast food joint is not as inexpensive and practical as it first appears to be. It eventually costs us in terms of our mental health. Examine your diet
There isn't a magic food that can cure depression. But how you feel can actually and significantly be impacted by what you put into your body.

When they stay away from processed meals, sugar, and preservatives, some people report feeling better and having more energy.

If you can, think about consulting a qualified nutritionist or doctor for advice.

A good place to start could be eating a diet high in lean meats, veggies, and grains. Limit stimulants like caffeine as much as possible. Also limit the intake of coffee, and soda, and depressants such as alcohol.

When depressed, it's a good idea to limit your intake of fat and sweets. But which foods can help treat depression?

What to eat to combat sadness naturally
How changing your diet might make you feel better or worse

Consuming fruits, nuts, and leafy greens can aid the body's ability to combat sadness. In fact, one study found that people who consume fewer fruits and vegetables are more prone to experience depression. Your thoughts and feelings may be directly impacted by what you consume. Make sure to consume a nutrient-rich, well-balanced diet. You can study your eating patterns with the aid of a dietician or nutritionist, who can also help you identify any nutrient deficiencies that might be causing your sadness.

Some foods may be particularly helpful when you are depressed, such as:

Fish: According to research, those who consumed a lot of fish in their diets were less likely to experience depressive symptoms.

15 Omega-3 fatty acids, which are abundant in fish, aid in the function of neurotransmitters like serotonin in the brain.
Nuts: One study found that people who ate walnuts were 26% less likely to experience depressive symptoms. Nuts are also a good source of omega-3 fats.
16
Probiotics: Growing evidence suggests a link between the health of the gut and the brain.
Yogurt, kefir, kimchi, and kombucha are examples of foods high in probiotics.
Foods to Combat Depression
Modify your thinking

As corny as it may sound, having positive thoughts can make you feel wonderful. Your mood genuinely is directly affected by your ideas. Consider consulting a therapist if you need help learning how to combat negativity.

Some foods, such as omega-3-rich walnuts, can enhance brain health and lessen depressive symptoms. Several studies also appear to support the idea that a Mediterranean diet, which emphasizes whole grains, seafood, vegetables, fruit, berries, nuts, and seeds, as well as the legendary cold-pressed olive oil, is an excellent means of treating depression.

Nutritionally speaking, the best ways to start treating depressive symptoms is to make sure you're getting enough:

- Vegetables (especially leaves that are green in color)

- Fruits

- Berries

- Nuts (including cashew)

- Seeds

Because a well-nourished body is better able to handle stress, physical illness, and stressful life events, these nutrient-rich meals help you feel better.

The traditional Mediterranean diet has been shown to be effective in treating depression, according to studies conducted by Professor Felice N. Jacka at the Department of Psychiatry at Deakin University, a prominent authority on diet and mental health.

A study found that moving from the western eating pattern to this naturally antidepressant diet helped 25% of depressed subjects recover.

It's crucial to concentrate on what not to consume when discussing nutrition and depression. While there is still much to learn about which nutrients can help prevent depressive symptoms, cutting back on refined sugar, which can be found in processed meals, soft drinks, and sweets, may be particularly helpful.

According to a research that looked at the diets of 5,000 men and was published online on July 27, 2020, those who consumed 87 grams or more of sugar per day (about three candy bars) had a 23% higher risk of being diagnosed with depression.

The relationship? Because the brain needs a steady supply of glucose, too much sugar can cause excessive emotional highs and lows.
When you're unhappy, you want to feel good, so you seek sugary treats that make you feel good rather than kale, but this could exacerbate your symptoms. To combat sugar cravings, keep wholesome snacks on hand at all times. You can therefore substitute a piece of fruit or a handful of almonds for sweets. This can aid in ending your sugar addiction and prevent depression from getting worse.

Adequate sleep

Sleep deprivation can make it difficult to obtain enough rest, and inadequate sleep can exacerbate depression.

How can you help? Make some lifestyle adjustments to start. Every day, go to bed and rise at the same hour. Avoid taking a sleep. Remove any sources of distraction from your bedroom, including the computer and TV. Your sleep may get better over time.
Depression can be naturally treated without medicine with sleep.
Better sleep leads to happier mood

It is real. Sleeping is another activity that helps lessen depressed symptoms and maintain your mood on a regular basis. Additionally, there are numerous free things you may do at home to develop sound sleeping habits. The most recent sleep study suggests that sleep can function as an overnight therapy, improving our ability to manage intense emotions.

How may getting more restful sleep help you combat depression?
Moreover, 90% of those who are depressed have trouble sleeping. You've probably seen that some depressed people sleep excessively while others don't get enough rest. Inadequate sleep can also raise the risk of both mild and severe depression. Have you ever observed, for instance, how a lack of sleep may make you exhausted and depressed? Also, it may be challenging to concentrate the day following a restless night.

Some depressive symptoms are present. It's a good thing that modifications to one will have an impact on the other. Better sleep will improve your ability to focus and control your emotions. The best part is that this method of treating depression is convenient, cost-free, and does not require the use of drugs.

The most effective sleeping aid
There are some great methods to help you enhance your sleep pattern, no matter how it now seems. Your depression symptoms will lessen as a natural result. The skills are the same whether you're sleeping too much or too little, and sleep is one of the finest medication-free depression treatments we have. There is a leading sleeping aid that is advised by therapists.

Establish a bedtime and a consistent wake-up time.
Hence, the best thing you can do to improve your sleep is to make the decision to get up and go to bed at the same time every day, including on the weekends. Set an alarm for 90 minutes before going to bed to begin your relaxing time. Going to bed when you don't feel exhausted is pointless.

Also, if you can't fall asleep and are lying in bed for more than 20 minutes, get out of bed and do something soothing until you fall asleep. then go back to bed. Your brain will begin to equate the bed with being awake if you stay up late in bed.

Check out these methods for enhancing sleep and lessening depression symptoms if you don't enjoy this sleep aid or feel it's too difficult to begin with:

- Locate an "opportunity" to sleep for 8 hours each night.

- The bedroom should be set at roughly 18 degrees.

- Before bed, take a hot bath or shower.

- At night, use mood lighting.

- Install software that reduces screen's blue LED light

- 2 hours before bedtime, no screens

- Have a bedroom that is really dark (or wear a sleeping mask)

- No coffee or caffeine after noon

- 90 minutes before going to bed and relax

Download our free treatment app if you want additional details about these sleep aids before you start making adjustments. For novices, it has a whole module on sleep that includes both theory and assignments.

Mood and sleep are closely related. Whether you have depression or not, getting too little of the former will inevitably have an impact on the latter. Make sure you practice what sleep specialists refer to as "excellent sleep hygiene" to promote your mental wellbeing.

This entails maintaining regular bedtimes and wake-up times, having a peaceful bedtime routine that doesn't involve staring at a screen, having a bedroom that is dark, quiet, and uncluttered, and so on.

It can be difficult to understand how depression and sleep are related. Not only is it believed that inadequate sleep contributes to the development of depression, but depression itself can result in inadequate sleep.

There are steps you may do to try to enhance the quality of your sleep, regardless of whether you have trouble falling asleep or staying asleep:

Prior to going to bed, give yourself some downtime. Relax and steer clear of stressful activities or thoughts.
Set an alarm for the same time each morning and go to bed at the same time every night.

Establish a regular bedtime routine

Put away your gadgets and try spending a short while reading a book. Furthermore, make an effort to spend some time outside every day, despite the temptation to close the blinds and stay indoors. Sleep cycles and circadian rhythms are greatly influenced by light2, therefore it may be more difficult to fall asleep at night when there is less sunlight.

Take on responsibilities.

When you're depressed, you might wish to withdraw from society and abdicate your duties at work and home. Don't. Maintaining an active lifestyle and taking on regular duties will help you fight depression. They help you feel grounded and accomplished.

It's okay if you can't handle full-time employment or education. Consider working part-time. If that seems excessive, think about volunteer work.

Challenge negative thoughts.

Cognitive behavioral therapy is one of the most widely used and successful approaches to treating depression (CBT). This type of psychotherapy is centered on recognizing destructive thought patterns and then changing them to more constructive ones. You can put some of these concepts into practice on your own in a variety of ways.

Changing your thought process is a big part of the battle against depression. When you're depressed, you automatically draw the worst conclusions. How to Spot Negative Thought
These ideas may occasionally be plainly audible, such as when you chastise or condemn yourself. Sometimes they are more subdued. You can catch yourself doing things like catastrophizing or thinking all or nothing.

Catastrophizing means constantly expecting the worse. When you conceive of things as either successes or failures with no room in between, you are said to have an all-or-nothing mindset. You can start developing some healthier options as you become more adept at seeing these cognitive habits.

Reorient Your Thinking
Consciously change your negative thoughts to positive ones whenever you catch yourself thinking one. For instance, instead of saying "This will never work," you might say something more encouraging like "Here are a few things I can try to get started." You can keep a more upbeat attitude by refocusing on your skills and capabilities.

CBT is a successful depression treatment that focuses on identifying and altering unfavorable thought patterns that fuel depressive symptoms. By becoming more conscious of your negative thoughts and changing them to more realistic and optimistic ones, you can try these techniques on your own.

How to Change Your Negative Thoughts
Take Control of Your Stress
A brain hormone called cortisol, which has been proven to be higher in those with depression, can be increased by stress.
19 Time management, meditation, and biofeedback training are just a few of the many stress-reduction techniques available.

Use logic as a natural depression cure the next time you're having a bad self-esteem moment. Even if you could think no one likes you, is there any solid proof of that? Even if you may feel the most worthless person on the earth, is it truly the case? You can eventually stop those negative thoughts before they spiral out of control with practice.

Before using supplements, consult your doctor."

The research for specific vitamins to treat depression is encouraging. They consist of SAMe, folic acid, and fish oil. But before we can be certain, further research must be conducted. Before beginning any supplement, always discuss with your doctor, especially if you're already on medicine..

Try something new.

You're stuck in a rut when you're depressed. Encourage yourself to try something new. Visit a gallery. Read a worn book while sitting on a park seat. Participate in a soup kitchen. Attend a language course.
Depression frequently saps your enthusiasm and drive to try new things. Making a list of potential items to try and checking them off one at a time might be useful. You might have to convince yourself to try them, and you could realize that you don't necessarily have the urge to pursue new things beyond your initial attempt.

Yet, with time you can discover something that piques your interest or gives you more drive. Since it's not always simple, think about setting the objective of trying at least one new thing per week. That could offer you something to look forward to and help you combat boredom.

When we challenge ourselves to accomplish something different, there are molecular changes in the brain. Dopamine, a brain neurotransmitter related to pleasure, enjoyment, and learning, is altered when you try something new.

Have fun

Make time for your favorite hobbies if you're feeling down. What if there is no longer any enjoyment? That is merely a depressive symptom. Regardless, you must continue to try.

You have to put effort into having enjoyment, as weird as it may sound. Even if they seem like a chore, schedule activities you formerly enjoyed. Continue to see movies. Continue having supper out with pals.

Keep drugs and alcohol to a minimum.

Substance usage is very common among sad people.

You could be more likely to turn to alcohol, marijuana, or other drugs to ease the symptoms of your depression.

It's unclear whether drug and alcohol abuse causes depression.

But persistent drug use can change how your brain works, exacerbate pre-existing mental health conditions, or even result in the development of new ones.

It's possible to lose the ability to appreciate life when you're depressed. You must rediscover how to do it.

Activities that are pleasant will ultimately feel enjoyable again. Even by itself, alcohol has depressing effects. The ability to overcome the blues depends on receiving a good night's sleep, which might be disrupted by drinking. Even though consuming alcohol might seem like a quick treatment for your problems, it can often make them far worse.

Also, it can weaken inhibitions, which could lead to risky behavior and poor judgment that could have long-term effects.

If you are taking any form of antidepressant, you shouldn't drink at all. Medication and alcohol don't mix well.

If you've been misusing alcohol or other substances and need help quitting, go to your doctor. You can possibly be suffering from a drinking or drug use disorder. You may require additional support as you go through the recovery process because withdrawal symptoms might momentarily exacerbate depressive symptoms. Mood disorders can result from substance use.

Can depression be treated without drugs or antidepressants?
Sure, there is a straightforward response to this query. It is, indeed. The majority of individuals are unaware that depression can be treated without medication at home. If they do, most people are unable to achieve it.

The truth is that you can overcome depression without the use of drugs, even to lessen depressive symptoms. Your symptoms might dramatically or completely subside if you make a few little lifestyle adjustments at home. No antidepressant drug is mentioned among the five therapies for depression that are introduced in this chapter.

Use meditation to prevent depression.
Occasionally, meditation can replace medication.
Regular meditation practice is another priceless tool you may use to alleviate depression naturally. You can recover from a depressed episode and avoid relapsing into one by regularly practicing meditation.

According to one study, 63.6% of the participants said daily meditation helped them overcome mental health crises and negative thinking.

Beyond enhancing mental health, meditation is a mind-body health practice that has many other advantages.

Consider meditation as mood maintenance. It can aid in improving your emotional management, identifying depression symptoms earlier, and preventing the progression of your symptoms.

Meditation essentially involves three simple steps:

- Put your attention on the here and now (for example by noticing your breathing).
- Try not to criticize what you discover.
- Bring your attention back to the task at hand whenever you find yourself becoming sidetracked by thoughts (which you will).

You can alleviate depression naturally by engaging in this excellent mental activity.

Depression and mindfulness meditation
Because mindfulness gives you the ability to manage the distressing negative thoughts sadness can bring, meditation is particularly useful at battling depression. Check out the video below if you have trouble controlling intrusive, unpleasant thoughts. The first illustrates how a depressive spiral can start with a single bad idea. In the second video, mindfulness-based practices are used to demonstrate how to halt this spiral early on.

How to break out of a negative mental cycle while experiencing sadness
Does meditation alter the way the brain is built?
While attempting to treat depression without medication, meditation can be helpful because it will probably improve how your brain processes intense emotions.

In 2007, Dr. Lukk Harp and his colleagues at the University of Toronto Mississauga in Canada set out to determine whether those who frequently meditated reacted to melancholy differently from those who didn't. They did, it turned out. Regular meditation practitioners used their brain's "present moment network" to cope with sadness. In other words, they were able to feel melancholy without getting caught up in it or escalating it with anxious thoughts.The "evaluation" network of the brain was utilized by the non-meditators. In other words, individuals became preoccupied with depressing ideas such "why do I feel this way?," "how can I stop this?", "there's something wrong," etc. These are some images of their brains:

Depression recurrence can be prevented and depressive symptoms can be reduced with mindfulness meditation. Regular meditation practice is unquestionably advised if you're looking for a holistic approach to treating depression without drugs.

How long does it take for meditation to reduce depression symptoms?
We don't really know yet is the best response that can be given. The precise mindfulness meditation dosage that will most successfully lower depression requires further study. But as of right present, everyone agrees on 10 to 30 minutes every day. That's a good beginning.

Don't know where to start while practicing meditation?
Not to worry. For that, an app exists. Our science-based, psychologist-developed depression software teaches you how to incorporate regular meditation into your drug-free treatment. You can begin your road

to a calmer, quieter mind by downloading whenever you're ready (it's completely free, forever).

5. Use brain stimulation to treat depression
An at-home method for treating depression that is both secure and effective

Transcranial direct current stimulation is a method of brain stimulation that can be used to treat depression without the use of drugs. Although brain stimulation has been used for years to treat depression, relatively few people are aware of this viable treatment option. First off, tDCS is a non-invasive neurmodulation technique that differs significantly from electric shock therapy in that the current used in tDCS is 400 times weaker.

It operates by delivering a low energy direct current waveform to the desired brain area. Instead of activating neurons, this low energy current alters the brain's plasticity and influences how likely they are to fire. Now that we have created a wireless headset that gives this mild electrical stimulation, you can use it at home to treat the symptoms of depression, just like it is used in clinics to effectively treat depression.

 The dorsolateral prefrontal cortex is the objective of the treatment, and electrodes are positioned high on the scalp. Reduced levels of activity in this region of the brain are linked to depressed symptoms such weariness, trouble sleeping, difficulty concentrating, and changes in appetite. The electrical current used in tDCS activates the DLPFC, reducing depression symptoms by activating brain activity there. By combining lifestyle modifications with an evidence-based treatment, you can avoid the negative side effects of antidepressant medication, such as weight gain and sleep issues. Here are a few additional advantages:

Major Depressive Disorder can be treated with a combination of behavior therapy and tDCS brain stimulation delivered through a portable headset.

There are fewer and less severe side effects than with antidepressants because it is a proven method for treating depression without drugs.

With the approach, 30% of participants totally beat depression. 71% report that within two weeks, at least half of their depression symptoms have vanished.

Depression is treatable in the comfort of your own home.

As you can see, there are a variety of drug-free alternatives to treating depression, and no single method is certain to be effective for everyone. There are other conventional therapies too.

Cut Back on Caffeine

Caffeine is a common ingredient in coffee, tea, soda, and even chocolate. Caffeine in moderation is acceptable in the morning if you love it, but stay away from it after late afternoon to prevent sleep disruption.

If you do have a tendency to rely on caffeine, try reducing your intake gradually to prevent unpleasant withdrawal symptoms. Instead of indulging your urge for soda or coffee, consider taking a little stroll around the block.

What You Should Know About Caffeine
Get Extra Vitamin D
There is some evidence that suggests depression may be exacerbated by a vitamin D deficiency.
3 Ask your doctor if you should consider taking a supplement if your food and lifestyle (such as sun exposure) aren't providing you with adequate vitamin D.

Certain nutrient deficiencies can play a role in depression symptoms. If you are having a difficult time spending enough time outdoors or if overcast weather conditions make it hard to get sunshine, a supplement may be useful.

Try Natural Remedies

There may be natural antidepressants that can help lessen the symptoms of depression, according to some study. Dietary supplements including St. John's Wort, S-adenosylmethionine (SAM-e), and 5-Hydroxytryptophan (5-HTP) may be worth a try for treating mild to moderate depression.

In the past, the same peak-x adulterant that caused eosinophilic-myalgic syndrome and over 300 fatalities in Japan was shown to be contaminating 5-HTP.
The U.S. Food and Drug Administration does not regulate dietary supplements, thus it is very important to utilize them with caution.
St. John's wort is more helpful than a placebo for reducing symptoms in those with mild to moderate depression, according to research.

Omega-3 fatty acids have also been investigated for their potential impact on depression. One 2015 study found that taking omega-3 supplements may help reduce symptoms of depression in both adults and children, although researchers are not entirely sure how or why.7

It has also been looked into how omega-3 fatty acids may affect depression. Although researchers are not completely certain how or why, one 2015 study found that consuming omega-3 supplements may help lessen depressive symptoms in both adults and children. 7

Even while natural treatments for depression can be effective, you should always speak with your doctor before using them. It doesn't automatically follow that something is safe just because it's advertised as natural and is available without a prescription.

A few of these natural antidepressants may also have undesirable side effects or interact negatively with other medications, and research on some of them is still unclear. For instance, combining St. John's wort with an SSRI like Prozac may result in serotonin syndrome, a side effect. 8 SAM-e

also raises the possibility of hypomania/mania in bipolar patients.
9\sRecap

Although some herbs and other supplements may function as natural antidepressants, this does not necessarily imply that they are risk-free, suitable for everyone, or free from adverse effects. Also, it's not always apparent whether these natural cures work, so always consult your doctor first.

Engage your spiritual side

Many people with depression find that religion may be a significant source of support, but you are under no need to join a church, synagogue, or mosque unless you so choose. Basic daily routines like meditation or adding to your list of gratitude can help boost mood and overall well-being.

Reduced stress and increased awareness of one's thoughts and behaviors are only two of the many positive consequences of meditation.

According to research, a therapy called mindfulness-based cognitive therapy (MBCT), which combines mindfulness meditation with cognitive behavioral therapy (CBT), can be effective in treating depression and preventing relapses in the future.

Research imply that various forms of mindfulness meditation can be helpful in the management of depression.

There are many various styles of meditation, but by following these steps, you can begin with a basic meditative exercise:

- Sit back and relax.
- Shut your eyes.
- respire normally.
- Pay attention to how your body feels when you breathe.
- Bring your focus back to your breathing whenever your thoughts stray.

You might want to add the following stress-relieving activities in your everyday routine:

Deep breathing can help you manage your worries better. Take a few minutes to slow your breathing and concentrate on your body right now.
Exercise is a terrific method to let off steam on a regular basis.
Progressive muscle relaxation: This technique entails consciously contracting all of the body's muscles, holding that tension for a number of counts, and then gradually releasing it until the muscles are completely relaxed.

You might be able to develop the ability to deliberately relax your body whenever you are feeling tight with frequent practice. It takes time and effort to develop stress management skills. Talk to your doctor or therapist about other strategies you might try to minimize the stress and your response to it.

Improve Your House or Workplace with Greenery
Indoor plants can improve the atmosphere in your house or place of business. It makes sense that "bringing the outdoors in" would assist enhance your mood because natural environments are linked to better mental well-being.

According to studies, adding indoor plants to your house or place of business can be beneficial in a number of ways, including:

Enhancing the workplace: Studies have shown that adding indoor plants to office areas increases worker contentment and concentration.
Lowering stress: According to a different study, taking care of indoor plants actively interacts with them and lowers both physical and mental stress.

Reducing anxiety and depression: According to research, pupils who spent the majority of their time at home during the COVID-19 pandemic had better mental health if they were exposed to more green plants. 24 The participants who were exposed to more greenery had reduced levels of despair and anxiety, even though nearly a third of them reported having moderate depressive symptoms.

Selecting particular plants could have added advantages. For instance, research indicates that the aroma of a lavender plant may promote calmness and relaxation. Greenery may be a terrific way to enhance your surroundings and possibly lift your mood, regardless of the kind of plants you select.

Take Care of Your Social Life

There are numerous reasons to seek out to friends and family when you're depressed rather than struggling on your own. Establish plans with family and friends and adhere to the dates. Join a club or enrol in a group activity, like a French class or a local dodgeball league.

Sign up for a support group.

Speaking with others who are facing same difficulties and experiences can be instructive and beneficial.
Plan your activities.
When you're depressed, having routines can be beneficial.
Make sure that your daily plan includes time for socializing. If it is a scheduled event, you are more likely to follow through.

A fantastic method to make new friends and widen your social circle is to get involved in a cause that you believe in.
The issue is that depression frequently leads to withdrawal, which further worsens feelings of loneliness and isolation. Even if you don't feel like going out or interacting with people, try reaching out in the method that feels most natural to you. Recruit a couple of your closest family members who can relate to what you are going through.

When you're depressed, doing the activities you used to like might not be as enjoyable, but leaving the house and spending time with people you care about can make you feel better.

Listen to Upbeat Music
It goes without saying that music can affect how you feel, so picking the proper tunes to listen to while you're feeling depressed may help you feel better.

According to research, those who are depressed may have a propensity to listen to songs that amplify their ruminating, melancholy, and emotion-focused coping.

Hence, instead of listening to depressing songs that make you want to cry, think about choosing music that make you feel better and are more uplifting.

Showing thankfulness People with depression have been proven to experience positive emotional effects by doing so. According to a study published in the March 2020 issue of NeuroImage, writing down the things in your life that you are grateful for can boost activity in the medial prefrontal cortex, a part of the brain that is frequently linked to depression.

You might be appreciative for something as uncomplicated as having all of your traffic lights turn green while driving or for someone holding the door for you as you approach the building.

Start a gratitude journal and write down instances of things that make you grateful. When you're feeling down, read through those entries for inspiration.

It's not necessary to write daily; some studies show that even writing only once a week might be beneficial.

Don't merely list the people and things you are grateful for; instead, attempt to explain why you are thankful for them and how they have improved your life.

Social connection
It is undeniable that social isolation raises a person's chance of developing depression and can exacerbate and prolong symptoms. Socializing is obviously more challenging when you're depressed. Joining an organization dedicated to a cause you are passionate about is one solution.

For instance, volunteering for a cause you care about can help you stay in touch with people on a regular basis, and your personal interest in the cause gives you an extra incentive to participate. Joining a team that competes in a sport you enjoy, like tennis, golf, or bowling, is another option.

CHAPTER FIVE

ANXIETY

What is anxiety?
A sensation of worry, dread, and unease is known as anxiety. You can start to perspire, become agitated and anxious, and experience rapid heartbeat. That can be a typical response to stress. You might have anxiety, for instance, when confronted with a challenging challenge at work, before taking a test, or before making a crucial decision. It may enable you to manage. You might feel more energized or able to concentrate if you're anxious. But for some with anxiety disorders, the terror can be incapacitating and last for a long time.

What are Anxiety disorders?
Conditions known as anxiety disorders are characterized by persistent anxiety that might deteriorate with time. The symptoms can interfere with daily activities such as job performance, schoolwork, and relationships.

What are the types of anxiety disorders?
There are several types of anxiety disorders, including:

Generalized anxiety Disorder(GAD). GAD patients worry about everyday matters like their health, finances, jobs, and families. Yet they have been worrying excessively for at least six months, and they worry virtually every day.

panic illness. Panic attacks occur in people with panic disorder. When there is no risk, these are brief but frequent episodes of extreme terror. The assaults start off abruptly and can linger for a few minutes or longer.
Phobias. Individuals who suffer from phobias have a strong fear of something even though it presents little or no real risk. They might be afraid of flying, spiders, crowded areas, or social situations (known as social anxiety).

What causes anxiety disorders?
Anxiety has an unidentified origin. Genetics, brain chemistry and biology, stress, and your surroundings are only a few possible contributing factors.

Who is susceptible to anxiety conditions?
The risk factors for various anxiety disorders can differ. For instance, GAD and phobias are more prevalent in women, yet both men and women experience social anxiety. The following are some universal risk factors for all varieties of anxiety disorders:

- Being shy or reticent in unfamiliar situations or when you meet new people are examples of certain personality traits.

- early childhood trauma or adulthood trauma

- Having anxiety or other mental illnesses runs in the family

- Many physical health issues, like thyroid issues or arrhythmia

What signs or symptoms indicate an anxiety disorder?
Different symptoms may be present depending on the type of anxiety illness. But they all combine some of the following:

- difficulty to control anxious thoughts or beliefs.
- They disrupt your regular life and give you a restless, nervous feeling.
- They persist and have the potential to develop worse with time.

Physical signs like shortness of breath, a racing or pounding heartbeat, inexplicable aches and pains, and dizziness
changes in behavior, such as refraining from routine tasks you used to perform
Caffeine, other beverages, and specific medications can exacerbate your symptoms.

How are anxiety disorders diagnosed?
Your doctor will inquire about your symptoms and medical background in order to diagnose any anxiety problems. To be sure that a separate health issue is not the source of your symptoms, you might also undergo a physical examination and lab tests.

You will have a psychological assessment if you don't have any further health issues. You might acquire one from your doctor, or you might be directed to a mental health specialist to get one.

What medications are used to treat anxiety disorders?
Psychotherapy (talk therapy), medications, or a combination of both are the primary therapies for anxiety disorders:

A form of psychotherapy called cognitive behavioral therapy (CBT) is frequently used to treat anxiety disorders. You learn many ways of thinking and acting with CBT. It can assist you in altering your response to situations that make you feel anxious and fearful.

Exposure treatment could be a part of it. This focuses on getting you to face your anxieties so you can do the things you had been putting off. Anti-anxiety medications and certain antidepressants are among the medications used to treat anxiety disorders. Certain types of anxiety disorders may respond better to some medications than others. To determine which medication is best for you, you should work closely with your healthcare practitioner. Before you can locate the proper medication, you might need to test a few different ones.

CHAPTER SIX

RELATIONSHIP BETWEEN ANXIETY AND DEPRESSION

Although anxiety and sadness are more closely related than you may imagine, anxiety is typically thought of as a high-energy condition and despair as a low-energy state. Anxiety is a common symptom of depression, and it may even reach the point where panic attacks occur. [1]

There is more to anxiety disorders than just regular trepidation and worry. They have the power to instill horrifying fear in people about topics that other people wouldn't even consider. Many individuals with anxiety disorders are completely aware of the irrationality of their ideas. Still, they are unable to stop them. They are plagued by thoughts of losing control inside. One of the entrances to sadness is this angst.

Why Are Anxiety and Depression Often Co-occurring?
It's a vicious cycle. When you feel anxious, you frequently think about your worries or problems. You regret doing it. You then feel like a failure. You start to feel depressed.

Anxiety and depression are two disorders with a complex relationship:

When there is an anxiety problem present, the likelihood of developing depression is significantly increased. Almost half of people who have significant depression also have severe, ongoing anxiety.
Individuals who are depressed frequently experience worry and anxiety. The two can readily lead to one another, with anxiety frequently coming before sadness.

Depression is most likely to strike those who have post-traumatic stress disorder (PTSD).
A person's struggle is frequently rooted in a biological propensity for both of these illnesses. More so than with depression, this seems to apply to anxiety disorders. Some folks are just worriers and pass it down.

Individuals who have an anxiety disorder should discuss their symptoms with a psychiatrist, therapist, or other healthcare provider. Avoid delaying treatment for an anxiety illness. Depression may be able to move in and take up residence in such people if it is not detected in time.

What Motivates Fear?
Even when there is no real threat, the fight-or-flight region in these people's brains activates for reasons that are currently only partially understood.

 Constant anxiousness is like being pursued by a predator who cannot be seen. There is always a persistent sense of threat. They are constantly on guard.

It's common to have uneasiness every now and then. People frequently experience anxiety when dealing with marital difficulties, workplace issues, impending important tests, or having to make a huge decision. Nevertheless, anxiety disorders go beyond momentary apprehension or fear. Anxiety does not go away for those with an anxiety condition. With time, it frequently gets worse to the point where people's daily functions are affected by their emotions.

Why Do People Become Depressed?
According to recent studies, a mix of genetic, biochemical, environmental, and psychological variables contribute to depression. Although it can happen at any age, it frequently starts in maturity. Depression in children and adolescents may manifest more as irritation than low mood, similar to many anxiety disorders.

Depression manifests as hopelessness, despair, and wrath by adulthood. Low energy levels make those who suffer from them frequently feel as though they cannot handle life's essential daily responsibilities and interpersonal relationships.

As was already mentioned, untreated anxiety disorders frequently result in depression.

What Signs of Anxiety and Depression Could Be Present?
The following characteristics could indicate either an anxiety condition or depression:

- irrational concerns or persistent feard

- physical signs such exhaustion, headaches, an irregular heartbeat, difficulty breathing, or stomach pain.

- having trouble falling or staying asleep.

- alterations in eating patterns, whether excessive or insufficient

- difficulty concentrating, remembering, or making judgments

- persistent dejection or sense of worthlessnes

- loss of regular interest in hobbies or activities

- being frequently exhausted and irritable

- inability to unwind and enjoy the present

- having panic attacks, which cause them to feel as though they are losing control

Depression is a dangerous disorder that, if addressed, could get worse over time. If you don't want to use prescription antidepressant medication, there are several natural remedies you might try. These techniques can be beneficial when used in conjunction with various therapies, such as psychotherapy and medicine.

SUMMARY

To determine the most effective course of action for treating your depression, speak with your doctor or therapist. Many lifestyle modifications, including eating a nutritious diet, exercising frequently, and getting adequate sleep, may help reduce your symptoms. Before using any supplements to treat depression, always see your doctor because they could have their own side effects or interact negatively with any medications you might be on.

Always treat depression symptoms seriously because they don't go away on their own. Don't try to manage your symptoms on your own, even while there are many things you can do to assist your mental health. Discuss some of the self-help techniques that could supplement your treatment with your doctor.

All the strategies to conquer anxiety and sadness are summarized below:
1) Moving around

2) Avoid proscastination

3) Doing things in parts instead of in whole

4) Positive Thoughts

5) Set Goals

6) Reward yourself

7) Having a Routine

8) Being Joyful

9) Listening to Music

10) Appreciate Nature

11) Socialize with others

12) Journaling

13) Try Something new

14) Volunteer to help others

15) Show Gratitude

16) Focus on Meditation

17) Good Diet

18) Avoid Drugs and alcohol

19) Get enough sleep

Acceptance

You can take a number of actions to navigate and manage depression. Little adjustments to your daily schedule, nutrition, and way of life can all have a good impact.

Your energy may be sapped by depression, leaving you drained and worn out. It may be tough to generate the will or energy to seek treatment as a result. You could regulate these emotions by making little lifestyle adjustments.

Little changes, large effects

A person may develop clinical depression if they experience persistent, profound sadness or a loss of interest in activities. This illness is also known as major depressive disorder.

There are, however, simple actions you can take to give yourself greater control over your life and enhance your sense of wellbeing.

Continue reading to discover how to apply these tactics in a way that makes sense for you.

Begin by going where you are.
Depression is quite typical. Millions of individuals are impacted by it, including some in your life. You might not be aware that they encounter comparable difficulties, feelings, and hurdles.

Being honest, accepting, and loving of yourself and what you're going through is essential for overcoming depression.

With this disease, every day is unique. It's critical to treat your mental health seriously and acknowledge that you won't always be where you are.

If you want to get some exercise, think about going for a block walk.. Exercise can seem like the last thing you'd want to do on days when you don't feel like getting out of bed. Yet, physical activity and exercise can assist to lessen depressive symptoms and increase vigor.

According to research, for some people, exercise can help with depressive symptoms just as well as prescription drugs. It might also aid in avoiding recurrent depressed episodes.

See whether you'd be willing to do the opposite of what your mood is asking you to do, like snuggling up in bed, even when you feel like you can't or have very little energy. Have a more modest objective for yourself, like going for a short walk around the block.

Be aware that tomorrow may not resemble today.
Day to day variations in internal feelings and ideas are possible. This can be recalled by maintaining a mood journal or documenting experiences.

If you had trouble getting out of bed or achieving your goals today, keep in mind that you still have tomorrow to try again.. Let yourself the grace to understand that not all days will be difficult. Try to look forward to tomorrow's fresh start.

. Instead of generalizing the whole, evaluate the components.
Recollections can be colored by painful feelings due to depression. You might realize that you're concentrating on issues that are challenging or seen as being ineffective.

Stop trying to generalize so much. Strive to focus on the positive. If it helps, make a list of the significant aspects of the occasion or day. You can keep track of your day's accomplishments and determine which activities you enjoyed.

You might be able to shift your focus to the specific parts that were useful by realizing how much weight you're putting to one thing rather than the total.

Take the opposite action to what your "depression voice" advises.
Your inner voice could discourage you from seeking self-help. You can learn to overcome it, though, if you can learn to recognize it.

Say to yourself, "You might be correct, but it'll be better than just sitting here another night," when you are unsure whether an activity will be enjoyable or worthwhile. You might realize quickly that the automatic idea isn't always useful.

Make realistic objectives
A long list of tasks may be so burdensome that you'd prefer not to take any action. Consider defining smaller goals instead of creating a big list of chores. Establishing and achieving these objectives can increase motivation and give a feeling of control and accomplishment.

Among the achievable objectives are:

Take out the trash instead of cleaning the house.
Sort the piles of laundry by color rather than doing the entire mound of
wash.
Just respond to any time-sensitive emails instead of emptying your entire
inbox.
Focus on another tiny task after completing the first one, then another. In
this manner, rather of an unfinished to-do list, you have a list of concrete
accomplishments.

Recognize your work.
All objectives are deserving of honor, and all accomplishments are cause for
celebration. Try your best to acknowledge when you reach a goal.

Recognizing your own accomplishments can be a very effective tool against
depression's harmful effects, even if you don't feel like throwing a party
with cake and confetti.

It may be especially effective to resist inappropriate speech and
overgeneralization with memories of a task well done.

Establishing a routine might be beneficial for you.
If your daily schedule is disrupted by depressive symptoms, creating a mild
regimen may give you a sense of control. These schedules don't have to
cover the whole day.

Concentrate on developing a loose but disciplined routine that will enable
you to maintain your daily pace.

Do something enjoyable...
You can feel so exhausted that you give up. In comparison to desired
emotions, it could feel stronger.

Attempt to fight back by doing something you enjoy or that has meaning for you. It might be singing, dancing, drawing, motorcycling, or playing an instrument.

Your mood or energy may improve as a result of engaging in meaningful activities, which may inspire you to carry on with beneficial activities that aid in managing symptoms.

Enjoy music-listening
According to research, listening to music is a fantastic approach to reduce depression symptoms and lift your mood. Also, it might enhance your capacity for receiving good feelings.

When music is performed in groups, like a band or musical ensemble, it may be very useful.

The same benefits can also be obtained by merely listening.

Take in the outdoors. A person's mood can be greatly influenced by time spent in nature.According to research, those who suffer from severe depression may benefit from taking walks in the outdoors.

Spending time outdoors may enhance mood and cognition while reducing the risk of mental health issues. On the direct impact of nature on people who are suffering from clinical depression, there is, however, little evidence.

Take a stroll through the trees at lunchtime or spend some time in your neighborhood park. Or schedule a weekend hike. While getting some sun, these activities might help you re-connect with nature.

Be with family and friends.
Face-to-face time can help wash away these tendencies. Depression can tempt you to withdraw from the people you love and trust.

Calls or video chats can be useful if you can't physically spend time together.

Try to keep in mind that these folks genuinely care about you. Don't give in to the urge to feel like a burden. Both of you probably need the interaction.

. Express your emotions through writing or journaling.
Think about keeping a journal or writing about your feelings. When the emotions subside, write about that as well. According to research, journaling can be an effective supplemental technique for treating mental health issues.

It can be easier to convey how you're feeling when you write your thoughts down. It can also assist you in tracking your daily symptoms and determining their origins.

. Do something completely different
You employ the same brain regions when performing the same task repeatedly.

According to research, trying new things might make you feel better overall and improve and strengthen your social connections.

Consider starting a new sport, enrolling in a creative class, or learning a new cooking skill to enjoy these advantages.

Volunteering is a fantastic way to accomplish both.
By volunteering and donating your time to someone or something else, you can kill two birds with one stone—spending time with others and learning something new.

Even though you might be accustomed to getting assistance from pals, your mental health might be enhanced more by reaching out and offering assistance.. Those who volunteer also benefit physically. One benefit of this is a reduced risk of hypertension.

You can use this to develop your gratitude.
By taking the time to express gratitude for what you have, whether it be a favorite hobby or something new, you may be able to improve your mental health.

According to research, being grateful can improve your mental health in general.

Furthermore, it can be particularly significant to express your thanks in writing, including in notes to other people.

Meditation can help you center your thoughts.
Depression symptoms can be prolonged by stress and anxiety. You may reduce your stress and bring more joy and harmony into your day by learning relaxing techniques.

According to research, engaging in activities like meditation, yoga, deep breathing, and journaling may enhance your sense of wellbeing and make you feel more a part of the world.

Do not overindulge in alcohol and drugs.
Drugs and alcohol are two substances that might prolong depressive symptoms.

On the other hand, those who struggle with addiction may display depressive symptoms.

If you wish to relieve your depression symptoms, you might want to reduce or stop using alcohol and other drugs.

Getting sufficient rest can also make a difference.

Sleep issues are typical with depression. You can have trouble sleeping or sleep too much. Both can exacerbate the symptoms of depression.

Sleep for a minimum of 8 hours each night. Strive to establish a regular sleeping schedule.

It can be beneficial to go to bed and wake up at the same time each day if you want to keep to a routine. You might feel more balanced and energised during the day if you get enough sleep.

Recognize the truth in your feelings
It could seem like a wise move to compartmentalize and suppress your emotions in order to deal with the challenging depression symptoms. However, this method is ultimately harmful and unsuccessful.

Recognize if you're having a bad day. When you become aware of and recognize your emotions, attempt to direct your attention toward taking part in constructive activities rather than dwelling on them. Seeing the ebb and flow of depressive symptoms can be instructive for both self-healing and hope.
Take into account medical therapy
Talking to a specialist about what you're going through could also be useful. Your family doctor might be able to recommend you to a therapist or other expert.

They can evaluate your symptoms and assist in creating an individualized clinical treatment plan for you. This could involve a range of choices, like medication and treatment.

It could take some time to find the best course of treatment for you, so be honest with your doctor or other healthcare provider about what is and isn't working. They'll collaborate with you to identify the finest choice.
As individuals get older, a lot of people experience mild to moderate depression episodes. Health problems and the death of a spouse, relative,

or friend are frequent causes that might result in persistent sadness and loss of enjoyment.

My Experience With Depression
A recovery tale is a complicated thing. It has numerous beginnings but no definitive finale. There is a lot more inaction than action, and the most of the drama and struggle occurs internally. Much of the time, the main figure stays hidden in the shadows, making it impossible to even see what's happening.

I first became depressed when I was about 8 years old. There are pictures of me wearing the worn-out brown jacket that I preferred to wear. My mother took some really lovely pictures, and several of them have me in gloomy shadows, looking as depressed as I possibly could.

She needed to focus about her own sadness. My typical memory of her at that time is of a couch-bound mother who frequently took naps. She diagnosed her sleep disorder as sleepkophasia, a term I have never been able to locate in a dictionary. After resting down for a while, snap! Totally sleeping In those days, no one brought up odd emotional issues or mental disease. On occasion, my parents described someone suffering a nervous breakdown as if they had passed away. There was no indication that my mother, much less me, needed assistance. Since I was a star student, independent, and impressive to professors for being so mature, no one worried about me.

The onset of migraines and growing levels of anxiety about school followed. I skipped numerous days, felt guilty as though I were pretending, and became fixated on all of my shortcomings. I was alone in my room for a long time. All Depression disappeared during my teen years. Emotions could be harmful. I couldn't possibly add to the barrage of irate and aggressive ones that were trembling the house. I therefore suppressed my emotions even more than I did when I was younger.

Nothing both within my house and outside of it bothered me. I showed almost no sign of reaction to anything, even while churning with fear and anguish.

When I finally cracked in my 20s, torrents of depression, anxiety, terror, obsessive love, and rage came pouring out. I visited a psychiatrist after having a panic episode for a week. In a three-hour marathon session, he assisted me in connecting my panic to terrifying incidents in my personal history. I was instantly healed, but I never saw him again. To do more would have been premature.

During a second crisis a few years later, I was finally able to see a psychiatrist again and had my first experience with Elavil. Yet, I was unsure of what it was. I took a stimulant in the morning to get me going and a sleep aid at night. I just used it briefly, got over the crisis, and kept going to therapy. For the following eight years, I continued to see psychiatrists in various places. Yet nobody brought up despair.

In a letter to the draft board during the Vietnam War, a psychiatrist used the term to describe my problem for the first time. Yet, I didn't receive care for that issue. In those days, therapy was still done in the Freudian tradition and focused mostly on family dynamics and conflict. Going deeper was facilitated by depression. Exploring the history helped me in many ways and was a huge help in understanding the difficulties of the present. Yet, depression persisted in various forms and returned frequently throughout the following few decades. I experienced ups and downs related to marriage, having kids, and a few different occupations, yet there were also incredibly joyful and prosperous periods.

My wife eventually asked that I seek treatment after my depression got to the point where it was too disruptive. So I did in the end. The 1990s were at hand. I began a twelve-year tour of medications that didn't accomplish very much once Prozac became available. Therapy didn't help either, despite the fact that two psychiatrists had helped me recognize some of my more harmful behavioral tendencies. Every aspect of my life was impacted by depression, making it more and more difficult to maintain a job and a family. The medications seemed to do nothing but numb my emotions, leaving me feeling removed from everyone and unaffected by stress. That was similar to having the pain signals muted. My body or brain no longer gave any indication that something might be wrong. Although I was "OK," my relationships and job continued to fail.

Strangely, despite having lived with depression for so many years, I didn't have a lot of knowledge about it. I initially believed that the issue was solely related to my low mood, lack of energy, and lack of motivation. As things deteriorated, I eventually began to read extensively about it.

When I discovered the full extent of depression and how ubiquitous it might be across the body and mind, I was astounded. I at last had a clear, complete understanding of what depression was.

That was a significant development since it allowed me to finally consider the likelihood of improving. I could see that I wasn't inherently useless, that there were causes for my inability to concentrate, and that this sickness was also to blame for the regular slurring of my speech and thought processes. After all, perhaps the proper care could result in important adjustments.

Yet there were still hazards up ahead. I developed an obsession with the notion that depression is a neurological condition. I researched various types of depression, as well as neuroscience and countless other topics. That was a wise move, but after a while I found myself focusing more on the word "Depression" than the specifics of my personal case of the sickness.

I questioned how many diagnostic subgroups I fell under. I most definitely had one or more anxiety problems. Maybe bipolar II is more appropriate for me than major depressive illness. How does dissociation fit in? I interpreted the research study's conclusions as a proclamation of my doom.

Knowing I had a "genuine" disease was consoling. I could not only refute any doubters on the reality of depression. I also had the residual uncertainty that I had any problems as a weapon against my internalized stigma. I had considered the possibility that I was faking my illness in order to escape reality and hide my own frailty. Here was evidence that my brain's chemistry, not my imagination, was what was causing my despair.

Neurobiology was completely out of my hands. I was unable to recover on my own. I had to be treated with medicine or other methods, such as ECT, by doctors. That meant that instead of placing my hopes in my own ability to improve, I was placing them in them.

I became certain that depression would never go away when the medications didn't help. The future was lost hope. My life would keep getting worse. Could it possibly result in suicide, as it did for some of my friends?

Fortunately, when I gained more knowledge, I paid attention to the professionals who had a far larger understanding of the reasons of the sickness. I understood from Mitcher Freed's review of the studies on depression that factors that may contribute to the condition include genetics, family history, traumatic experiences, stress, and the malfunction of numerous bodily systems. No one was able to isolate a single cause or reduce it to a handful of neurotransmitters.

So I went back to the beginning and paid much closer attention to the specific symptoms I was experiencing. I studied the small nuances of daily life and realized that I had to take the initiative in my own healing. When it had any effect at all, medication performed a small part in easing the worst symptoms. I was able to work on the emotional and relationship effects and try to straighten out the aspects of my life I had some control over because of that small sense of relief.

I was adamant about ending the futility of depression. I resumed my psychotherapy and also explored a variety of self-help techniques. Many of them failed completely, yet despite setbacks, something inside of me drove me to keep trying.

Because I know that the loneliness will pass and that I can talk myself out of feeling lonely when I am not actually alone, I push myself to spend more time with my friends.

I consume all things swoon-worthy. I play along by pretending to be one of the characters, which causes me to experience their emotions rather than my own (or preventing myself from feeling). I sing along to Taylor Swift from the past. Because what could be more lovely than a summer romance involving Chevy trucks and Tim McGraw in a little country town? And even though I occasionally let my homework slide, I always force myself to put in some effort. In essence, I make myself live my life because, well, it's my life and I don't want to spend it feeling lonely when I'm not and numb when I might be amazing. Because of my depression, I do experience such feelings far more frequently than I would like, yet I still have to deal with them.

I will always experience depression since it is an illness.

I am who I am and my depression is a part of that.

Most importantly, I want to live this life since I only have one to live. Even if at times my despair makes me want to end my life, I stubbornly refuse.

My attempt to write about my experience with depression was one of the most significant ones. One of the ways I learn new things is by writing, but for years I had avoided doing it due to a strong fear. I now see that the underlying cause of my impasse was my attempt to write about topics other than despair. Writing came effortlessly after I was able to tackle that head-on.

The ideal media turned out to be blogging. Even when I felt miserable, it was bearable. I received a kind of support from the internet depression community that I had never experienced before. Leaving my high-stress job, which I was doing less and less successfully, was another crucial move. A profound sensation of vigor was restored when that ongoing stress was lifted. Following all of this, recuperation eventually began. I was caught off guard by it, and for a while I had my doubts that it would endure. But deep down, something had shifted. I started to believe in myself once more, and the inner feeling of worthlessness vanished.

I had discovered a genuinely fulfilling reason for writing, as well as the motivation and humor to do what I wanted to do. I was able to reclaim my consciousness and emotional presence so that I could rejoin my family as the visible father and husband.

Setbacks occur, as anyone who has struggled with depression their entire life will attest to. No easy happy conclusion exists. Yet if you're fortunate, an inner change takes place, and the new normal is a good existence as opposed to depression.

Considering that I am the author of my own life, I prefer to use a semicolon rather than a period whenever my melancholy urges me to do otherwise.

Hence, my depression impacts my life in this manner. That's how I handle it. I will, whether you like it or not.

READ MORE
Can You Use Turmeric to Help Treat Depression?
Medically reviewed by Karen Cross, FNP, MSN
Turmeric contains an active phytochemical, curcumin, which is an antioxidant and anti-inflammatory. Research has found that curcumin has the potential...